SUPER EASY DIABETIC COOKBOOK FOR BEGINNERS

Delicious & Simple Diabetic Recipes: A Beginner's Guide to Healthy Cooking

Dr Lily Morgan

COPYRIGHT PAGE

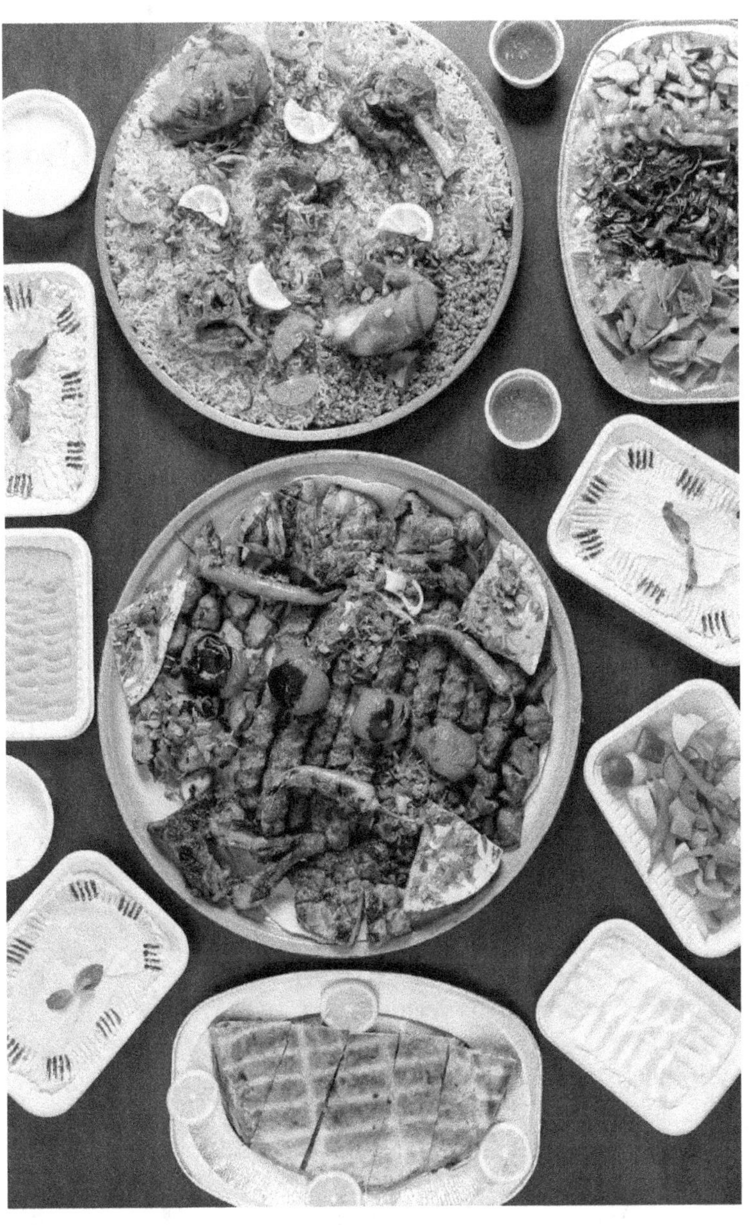

TABLE OF CONTENTS

Chapter 3: Lunch Recipes 37

Chapter 4: Dinner Recipes 51

Chapter 5: Snacks and Appetizers 66

INTRODUCTION

 elcome to the Super Easy Diabetic Cookbook, a comprehensive guide designed specifically for beginners who are looking to manage their diabetes through simple and delicious recipes. In this introductory chapter, we will explore the importance of a healthy diet in diabetes management and provide you with essential information to embark on your culinary journey.

Understanding Diabetes and Diet

Diabetes is a chronic condition that affects the body's ability to regulate blood sugar levels. It requires careful management, and one of the most crucial aspects is maintaining a balanced and nutritious diet. Understanding the relationship between diabetes and diet is essential for effectively managing the condition and promoting overall well-being.

In this section, we will delve into the various types of diabetes, including type 1, type 2, and gestational diabetes.

We will explain how these types differ and the impact they have on the body's insulin production and utilization. Additionally, we will discuss the role of diet in managing diabetes, highlighting the importance of portion control, carbohydrate counting, and the glycemic index.

Tips for Managing Diabetes Through Nutrition

When it comes to managing diabetes, making informed dietary choices is key. This section will provide you with practical tips and strategies to help you navigate your food choices and create a healthy eating plan tailored to your specific needs. We will cover topics such as:

The importance of meal planning: Learn how to structure your meals and snacks throughout the day to maintain stable blood sugar levels and prevent spikes or crashes.

Choosing the right carbohydrates: Discover the difference between simple and complex carbohydrates and how they affect your blood sugar. We will guide you in selecting the best sources of carbohydrates to incorporate into your diet.

Incorporating lean proteins: Explore the benefits of lean proteins and how they can contribute to satiety, muscle health, and blood sugar management. We will provide you with a variety of protein options suitable for a diabetic-friendly diet.

Emphasizing healthy fats: Understand the role of fats in your diet and learn to differentiate between good and bad fats. Discover sources of healthy fats that can promote heart health and overall well-being.

Including plenty of fruits and vegetables: Discover the wealth of nutrients found in fruits and vegetables and learn how to incorporate them into your meals. We will discuss portion sizes, cooking methods, and creative ways to make these nutrient powerhouses a central part of your diet.

Kitchen Tools and Ingredients

Equipping your kitchen with the right tools and ingredients can make your cooking experience more enjoyable and efficient. In this section, we will provide you with a list of essential kitchen tools that will help you prepare the recipes in this cookbook with ease. From measuring cups and spoons to food scales and blenders, we will guide you in assembling a well-equipped kitchen.

Furthermore, we will outline the essential ingredients you should have on hand for diabetic-friendly cooking. These pantry staples will form the foundation of your meals, providing you with a wide range of flavors and nutrients. We will emphasize the importance of reading food labels to make informed choices and identify hidden sugars or unhealthy additives.

Chapter 1: 30-Day Meal Plan

Week 1:

Day 1:

Breakfast: Avocado and Egg Breakfast Wrap

Lunch: Grilled Chicken Salad with Lemon Vinaigrette

Dinner: Baked Salmon with Roasted Vegetables

Snack: Guacamole with Veggie Sticks

Dessert: Mixed Berry Crisp

Beverage: Green Smoothie with Spinach and Apple

Day 2:

Breakfast: Blueberry Almond Overnight Oats

Lunch: Quinoa and Black Bean Salad

Dinner: Chicken and Vegetable Stir-Fry

Snack: Oven-Baked Sweet Potato Fries

Dessert: Sugar-Free Chocolate Mousse

Beverage: Iced Raspberry Tea

Day 3:

Breakfast: Spinach and Mushroom Frittata

Lunch: Turkey and Avocado Wrap

Dinner: Turkey Meatballs with Zucchini Noodles

Snack: Spicy Roasted Chickpeas

Dessert: Baked Apples with Cinnamon and Walnuts

Beverage: Cucumber and Mint Infused Water

Day 4:

Breakfast: Cinnamon Apple Quinoa Bowl

Lunch: Cauliflower Fried Rice

Dinner: Stuffed Bell Peppers with Quinoa and Ground Turkey

Snack: Greek Yogurt Dip with Fresh Veggies

Dessert: Greek Yogurt Popsicles

Beverage: Homemade Sugar-Free Lemonade

Day 5:

Breakfast: Greek Yogurt Parfait with Berries

Lunch: Tuna Salad Lettuce Wraps

Dinner: Baked Cod with Lemon and Herbs

Snack: Tomato and Mozzarella Skewers

Dessert: Almond Flour Chocolate Chip Cookies

Beverage: Almond Milk Latte

Day 6:

Breakfast: Vegetable and Egg Scramble

Lunch: Lentil Soup with Vegetables

Dinner: Beef and Broccoli Skillet

Snack: Baked Parmesan Zucchini Chips

Dessert: Fresh Fruit Salad with Citrus Dressing

Beverage: Strawberry Banana Smoothie

Day 7:

Breakfast: Whole Wheat Pancakes with Sugar-Free Maple Syrup

Lunch: Mediterranean Chickpea Salad

Dinner: Eggplant Parmesan with Whole Wheat Pasta

Snack: Hummus with Whole Wheat Pita Bread

Dessert: Pumpkin Spice Chia Pudding

Beverage: Coconut Water Electrolyte Drink

Week 2:

Day 8:

Breakfast: Smoked Salmon and Cream Cheese Bagel

Lunch: Greek Chicken Pita Pocket

Dinner: Grilled Shrimp with Garlic and Herbs

Snack: Caprese Salad Skewers

Dessert: Peanut Butter Energy Balls

Beverage: Sparkling Water with Citrus Slices

Day 9:

Breakfast: Banana Walnut Smoothie

Lunch: Caprese Skewers with Balsamic Glaze

Dinner: Vegetarian Chili with Quinoa

Snack: Cottage Cheese and Fresh Berries

Dessert: Lemon Poppy Seed Muffins (Sugar-Free)

Beverage: Chai Tea with Almond Milk

Day 10:

Breakfast: Veggie Breakfast Burrito

Lunch: Shrimp and Veggie Stir-Fry

Dinner: Lemon Herb Grilled Chicken Breast

Snack: Antipasto Skewers with Olives and Cheese

Dessert: Berry Parfait with Greek Yogurt

Beverage: Detox Water with Lemon and Ginger

Day 11:

Breakfast: Avocado and Egg Breakfast Wrap

Lunch: Grilled Chicken Salad with Lemon Vinaigrette

Dinner: Baked Salmon with Roasted Vegetables

Snack: Guacamole with Veggie Sticks

Dessert: Mixed Berry Crisp

Beverage: Green Smoothie with Spinach and Apple

Day 12:

Breakfast: Blueberry Almond Overnight Oats

Lunch: Quinoa and Black Bean Salad

Dinner: Chicken and Vegetable Stir-Fry

Snack: Oven-Baked Sweet Potato Fries

Dessert: Sugar-Free Chocolate Mousse

Beverage: Iced Raspberry Tea

Day 13:

Breakfast: Spinach and Mushroom Frittata

Lunch: Turkey and Avocado Wrap

Dinner: Turkey Meatballs with Zucchini Noodles

Snack: Spicy Roasted Chickpeas

Dessert: Baked Apples with Cinnamon and Walnuts

Beverage: Cucumber and Mint Infused Water

Day 14:

Breakfast: Cinnamon Apple Quinoa Bowl

Lunch: Cauliflower Fried Rice

Dinner: Stuffed Bell Peppers with Quinoa and Ground Turkey

Snack: Greek Yogurt Dip with Fresh Veggies

Dessert: Greek Yogurt Popsicles

Beverage: Homemade Sugar-Free Lemonade

Week 3:

Day 15:

Breakfast: Greek Yogurt Parfait with Berries

Lunch: Tuna Salad Lettuce Wraps

Dinner: Baked Cod with Lemon and Herbs

Snack: Tomato and Mozzarella Skewers

Dessert: Almond Flour Chocolate Chip Cookies

Beverage: Almond Milk Latte

Day 16:

Breakfast: Vegetable and Egg Scramble

Lunch: Lentil Soup with Vegetables

Dinner: Beef and Broccoli Skillet

Snack: Baked Parmesan Zucchini Chips

Dessert: Fresh Fruit Salad with Citrus Dressing

Beverage: Strawberry Banana Smoothie

Day 17:

Breakfast: Whole Wheat Pancakes with Sugar-Free Maple
Syrup

Lunch: Mediterranean Chickpea Salad

Dinner: Eggplant Parmesan with Whole Wheat Pasta

Snack: Hummus with Whole Wheat Pita Bread

Dessert: Pumpkin Spice Chia Pudding

Beverage: Coconut Water Electrolyte Drink

Day 18:

Breakfast: Smoked Salmon and Cream Cheese Bagel

Lunch: Greek Chicken Pita Pocket

Dinner: Grilled Shrimp with Garlic and Herbs

Snack: Caprese Salad Skewers

Dessert: Peanut Butter Energy Balls

Beverage: Sparkling Water with Citrus Slices

Day 19:

Breakfast: Banana Walnut Smoothie

Lunch: Caprese Skewers with Balsamic Glaze

Dinner: Vegetarian Chili with Quinoa

Snack: Cottage Cheese and Fresh Berries

Dessert: Lemon Poppy Seed Muffins (Sugar-Free)

Beverage: Chai Tea with Almond Milk

Day 20:

Breakfast: Veggie Breakfast Burrito

Lunch: Shrimp and Veggie Stir-Fry

Dinner: Lemon Herb Grilled Chicken Breast

Snack: Antipasto Skewers with Olives and Cheese

Dessert: Berry Parfait with Greek Yogurt

Beverage: Detox Water with Lemon and Ginger

Day 21:

Breakfast: Avocado and Egg Breakfast Wrap

Lunch: Grilled Chicken Salad with Lemon Vinaigrette

Dinner: Baked Salmon with Roasted Vegetables

Snack: Guacamole with Veggie Sticks

Dessert: Mixed Berry Crisp

Beverage: Green Smoothie with Spinach and Apple

Week 4:

Day 22:

Breakfast: Blueberry Almond Overnight Oats

Lunch: Quinoa and Black Bean Salad

Dinner: Chicken and Vegetable Stir-Fry

Snack: Oven-Baked Sweet Potato Fries

Dessert: Sugar-Free Chocolate Mousse

Beverage: Iced Raspberry Tea

Day 23:

Breakfast: Spinach and Mushroom Frittata

Lunch: Turkey and Avocado Wrap

Dinner: Turkey Meatballs with Zucchini Noodles

Snack: Spicy Roasted Chickpeas

Dessert: Baked Apples with Cinnamon and Walnuts

Beverage: Cucumber and Mint Infused Water

Day 24:

Breakfast: Cinnamon Apple Quinoa Bowl

Lunch: Cauliflower Fried Rice

Dinner: Stuffed Bell Peppers with Quinoa and Ground Turkey

Snack: Greek Yogurt Dip with Fresh Veggies

Dessert: Greek Yogurt Popsicles

Beverage: Homemade Sugar-Free Lemonade

Day 25:

Breakfast: Greek Yogurt Parfait with Berries

Lunch: Tuna Salad Lettuce Wraps

Dinner: Baked Cod with Lemon and Herbs

Snack: Tomato and Mozzarella Skewers

Dessert: Almond Flour Chocolate Chip Cookies

Beverage: Almond Milk Latte

Day 26:

Breakfast: Vegetable and Egg Scramble

Lunch: Lentil Soup with Vegetables

Dinner: Beef and Broccoli Skillet

Snack: Baked Parmesan Zucchini Chips

Dessert: Fresh Fruit Salad with Citrus Dressing

Beverage: Strawberry Banana Smoothie

Day 27:

Breakfast: Whole Wheat Pancakes with Sugar-Free Maple Syrup

Lunch: Mediterranean Chickpea Salad

Dinner: Eggplant Parmesan with Whole Wheat Pasta

Snack: Hummus with Whole Wheat Pita Bread

Dessert: Pumpkin Spice Chia Pudding

Beverage: Coconut Water Electrolyte Drink

Day 28:

Breakfast: Smoked Salmon and Cream Cheese Bagel

Lunch: Greek Chicken Pita Pocket

Dinner: Grilled Shrimp with Garlic and Herbs

Snack: Caprese Salad Skewers

Dessert: Peanut Butter Energy Balls

Beverage: Sparkling Water with Citrus Slices

Day 29:

Breakfast: Banana Walnut Smoothie

Lunch: Caprese Skewers with Balsamic Glaze

Dinner: Vegetarian Chili with Quinoa

Snack: Cottage Cheese and Fresh Berries

Dessert: Lemon Poppy Seed Muffins (Sugar-Free)

Beverage: Chai Tea with Almond Milk

Day 30:

Breakfast: Veggie Breakfast Burrito

Lunch: Shrimp and Veggie Stir-Fry

Dinner: Lemon Herb Grilled Chicken Breast

Snack: Antipasto Skewers with Olives and Cheese

Dessert: Berry Parfait with Greek Yogurt

Beverage: Detox Water with Lemon and Ginger

Chapter 2: Breakfast Recipes

In this chapter, we will explore a delightful array of breakfast recipes that are not only delicious but also suitable for individuals managing diabetes. These recipes are designed to provide a balance of nutrients, flavors, and textures to kickstart your day on a healthy note. So, let's dive into the scrumptious world of breakfast!

Avocado and Egg Breakfast Wrap

Ingredients:

- 1 whole wheat tortilla
- 1 ripe avocado, mashed
- 2 eggs, scrambled
- Salt and pepper to taste
- Salsa or hot sauce (optional)

Instructions:

1. Heat a non-stick pan over medium heat and scramble the eggs until cooked through. Season with salt and pepper.

2. Warm the tortilla in a separate pan or microwave for a few seconds.

3. Spread the mashed avocado evenly on the tortilla.

4. Place the scrambled eggs on top of the avocado.

5. Add salsa or hot sauce for extra flavor, if desired.

6. Roll up the tortilla tightly, securing it with a toothpick if needed.

7. Serve warm and enjoy this satisfying Avocado and Egg Breakfast Wrap.

Blueberry Almond Overnight Oats

Ingredients:

- 1/2 cup rolled oats
- 1/2 cup unsweetened almond milk
- 1/4 cup fresh blueberries
- 1 tablespoon almond butter
- 1 tablespoon chia seeds
- 1 teaspoon honey or sweetener of choice (optional)
- Sliced almonds for garnish

Instructions:

1. In a mason jar or container with a lid, combine the rolled oats, almond milk, blueberries, almond butter, chia seeds, and sweetener if using. Stir well to ensure everything is mixed thoroughly.

2. Seal the jar or container and refrigerate overnight or for at least 6 hours.

3. When ready to eat, give the mixture a good stir and top with sliced almonds.

4. Enjoy the delightful and nutritious Blueberry Almond Overnight Oats cold straight from the fridge.

Spinach and Mushroom Frittata

Ingredients:

- 4 eggs
- 1 cup fresh spinach, chopped
- 1/2 cup mushrooms, sliced
- 1/4 cup onion, finely chopped
- 1/4 cup low-fat feta cheese, crumbled
- Salt and pepper to taste
- Cooking spray or olive oil for greasing the pan

Instructions:

1. Preheat the oven to 350°F (175°C).
2. In a bowl, whisk the eggs until well beaten. Season with salt and pepper.
3. Heat a non-stick, oven-safe skillet over medium heat and lightly coat it with cooking spray or olive oil.
4. Sauté the onions and mushrooms until softened, then add the chopped spinach and cook until wilted.
5. Pour the beaten eggs into the skillet, evenly distributing the vegetables.
6. Sprinkle the crumbled feta cheese on top.
7. Transfer the skillet to the preheated oven and bake for 12-15 minutes, or until the eggs are set and slightly golden.
8. Remove from the oven and allow it to cool for a few minutes before slicing.
9. Serve a slice of this delicious Spinach and Mushroom Frittata with a side of fresh salad or whole grain toast.

Cinnamon Apple Quinoa Bowl

Ingredients:

- 1/2 cup cooked quinoa
- 1 small apple, diced
- 1 tablespoon chopped almonds or walnuts
- 1 teaspoon cinnamon
- 1/2 cup unsweetened almond milk
- 1 teaspoon honey or sweetener of choice (optional)

Instructions:

1. In a bowl, combine the cooked quinoa, diced apple, chopped almonds or walnuts, cinnamon, almond milk, and sweetener if desired. Mix well.
2. Microwave the mixture for 1-2 minutes or heat it on the stovetop until warm.
3. Stir again and let it sit for a few minutes to allow the flavors to meld.
4. Enjoy the cozy and nutritious Cinnamon Apple Quinoa Bowl as a comforting breakfast option.

Greek Yogurt Parfait with Berries

Ingredients:

- 1 cup plain Greek yogurt
- 1/2 cup mixed berries (strawberries, blueberries, raspberries)
- 2 tablespoons granola (look for sugar-free or low-sugar options)
- 1 teaspoon honey or sweetener of choice (optional)

Instructions:

1. In a glass or bowl, layer half of the Greek yogurt at the bottom.
2. Add half of the mixed berries on top of the yogurt.
3. Sprinkle a tablespoon of granola over the berries.
4. Repeat the layers with the remaining yogurt, berries, and granola.
5. Drizzle with honey or sweetener if desired.
6. Savor the delightful combination of creamy Greek yogurt, fresh berries, and crunchy granola in this Greek Yogurt Parfait.

Vegetable and Egg Scramble

Ingredients:

- 2 eggs
- 1/4 cup bell peppers, diced
- 1/4 cup zucchini, diced
- 1/4 cup cherry tomatoes, halved
- 1/4 cup onion, chopped
- Salt and pepper to taste
- Cooking spray or olive oil for greasing the pan

Instructions:

1. Heat a non-stick pan over medium heat and lightly coat it with cooking spray or olive oil.
2. Sauté the bell peppers, zucchini, cherry tomatoes, and onion until they are tender.
3. In a separate bowl, whisk the eggs and season with salt and pepper.
4. Pour the beaten eggs into the pan with the sautéed vegetables.
5. Continuously stir the mixture until the eggs are fully cooked and scrambled.

6. Transfer the Vegetable and Egg Scramble to a plate
    and serve hot.

Whole Wheat Pancakes with Sugar-Free Maple Syrup

Ingredients:

- 1 cup whole wheat flour
- 1 tablespoon baking powder
- 1/2 teaspoon cinnamon
- 1/4 teaspoon salt
- 1 cup unsweetened almond milk
- 1 egg
- 1 tablespoon olive oil or melted coconut oil
- Sugar-free maple syrup for topping

Instructions:

1. In a mixing bowl, whisk together the whole wheat
    flour, baking powder, cinnamon, and salt.
2. In a separate bowl, whisk the almond milk, egg, and
    oil until well combined.

3. Pour the wet ingredients into the dry ingredients and
    stir until just combined. Do not overmix; a few
    lumps are okay.

4. Heat a non-stick skillet or griddle over medium heat
    and lightly grease it with cooking spray or oil.

5. Pour 1/4 cup of batter onto the skillet for each
    pancake. Cook until bubbles form on the surface,
    then flip and cook for another 1-2 minutes until
    golden brown.

6. Remove the pancakes from the skillet and keep
    them warm.

7. Serve the Whole Wheat Pancakes with a drizzle of
    sugar-free maple syrup for a delightful and guilt-
    free breakfast treat.

Smoked Salmon and Cream Cheese Bagel

Ingredients:

- 1 whole wheat bagel, sliced and toasted
- 2 ounces smoked salmon
- 2 tablespoons low-fat cream cheese
- Fresh dill or chives for garnish

- Lemon wedges (optional)

Instructions:

1. Spread the cream cheese evenly on each half of the toasted bagel.
2. Place the smoked salmon on top of the cream cheese.
3. Garnish with fresh dill or chives for added flavor and visual appeal.
4. Squeeze lemon juice over the salmon, if desired.
5. Enjoy this classic and protein-packed Smoked Salmon and Cream Cheese Bagel as a filling breakfast option.

Banana Walnut Smoothie

Ingredients:

- 1 ripe banana
- 1 cup unsweetened almond milk
- 1 tablespoon almond butter
- 1 tablespoon ground flaxseeds
- 1/4 teaspoon vanilla extract
- 1/4 teaspoon cinnamon

- 1/4 cup crushed ice (optional)
- 1 tablespoon chopped walnuts for garnish

Instructions:

1. In a blender, combine the ripe banana, almond milk, almond butter, ground flaxseeds, vanilla extract, cinnamon, and crushed ice if using.
2. Blend until smooth and creamy.
3. Pour the smoothie into a glass and garnish with chopped walnuts.
4. Sip on the refreshing and nutritious Banana Walnut Smoothie to fuel your day.

Veggie Breakfast Burrito

Ingredients:

- 1 whole wheat tortilla
- 2 eggs, scrambled
- 1/4 cup bell peppers, diced
- 1/4 cup onion, chopped
- 1/4 cup black beans, drained and rinsed
- 1/4 cup shredded low-fat cheddar cheese
- Salt and pepper to taste

- Salsa or hot sauce (optional)
- Cooking spray or olive oil for greasing the pan

Instructions:

1. Heat a non-stick pan over medium heat and lightly coat it with cooking spray or olive oil.
2. Sauté the bell peppers and onion until they are tender.
3. Add the scrambled eggs and black beans to the pan, and cook until the eggs are fully cooked.
4. Season with salt and pepper.
5. Warm the whole wheat tortilla in a separate pan or microwave for a few seconds.
6. Place the scrambled eggs, vegetables, and black beans on the tortilla.
7. Sprinkle the shredded cheddar cheese on top.
8. Add salsa or hot sauce for an extra kick, if desired.
9. Roll up the tortilla tightly, securing it with a toothpick if needed.
10. Serve warm and relish the flavors of this wholesome Veggie Breakfast Burrito.

Chapter 3: Lunch Recipes

In this chapter, we will explore a variety of delicious and healthy lunch recipes that are perfect for individuals with diabetes. These recipes are designed to provide you with essential nutrients while keeping your blood sugar levels stable. Let's dive in and discover the flavors of these satisfying lunch options.

Grilled Chicken Salad with Lemon Vinaigrette

Ingredients:

- 2 boneless, skinless chicken breasts
- 4 cups mixed salad greens
- 1 cucumber, sliced
- 1 cup cherry tomatoes, halved
- 1/4 red onion, thinly sliced
- 1/4 cup sliced almonds
- Juice of 1 lemon
- 2 tablespoons olive oil
- 1 clove garlic, minced

- Salt and pepper to taste

Instructions:

1. Preheat the grill to medium-high heat.
2. Season the chicken breasts with salt and pepper.
3. Grill the chicken for about 6-8 minutes per side or until cooked through. Let it rest for a few minutes, then slice it into strips.
4. In a large bowl, combine the salad greens, cucumber, cherry tomatoes, red onion, and sliced almonds.
5. In a small bowl, whisk together the lemon juice, olive oil, minced garlic, salt, and pepper to make the vinaigrette.
6. Pour the lemon vinaigrette over the salad and toss to coat.
7. Divide the salad into plates and top with the grilled chicken slices.
8. Enjoy this refreshing and protein-packed grilled chicken salad.

Quinoa and Black Bean Salad

Ingredients:

- 1 cup cooked quinoa
- 1 cup canned black beans, rinsed and drained
- 1 red bell pepper, diced
- 1/2 cup corn kernels
- 1/4 cup chopped fresh cilantro
- 2 green onions, thinly sliced
- Juice of 1 lime
- 2 tablespoons olive oil
- 1 teaspoon cumin
- Salt and pepper to taste

Instructions:

1. In a large bowl, combine the cooked quinoa, black beans, red bell pepper, corn kernels, chopped cilantro, and sliced green onions.
2. In a small bowl, whisk together the lime juice, olive oil, cumin, salt, and pepper.
3. Pour the dressing over the quinoa and black bean mixture. Toss to combine.

4. Let the salad sit for about 15 minutes to allow the
    flavors to meld together.

5. Serve this colorful and nutritious quinoa and black
    bean salad as a refreshing lunch option.

Turkey and Avocado Wrap

Ingredients:

- 4 whole wheat tortillas
- 8 slices turkey breast
- 1 avocado, sliced
- 1/2 cup baby spinach leaves
- 1/4 cup diced tomatoes
- 2 tablespoons Greek yogurt
- 1 tablespoon Dijon mustard
- Salt and pepper to taste

Instructions:

1. Lay out the whole wheat tortillas on a clean surface.

2. Spread the Greek yogurt and Dijon mustard evenly
    on each tortilla.

3. Place two slices of turkey breast on each tortilla.

4. Top with avocado slices, baby spinach leaves, and diced tomatoes.

5. Season with salt and pepper.

6. Roll up the tortillas tightly, tucking in the sides as you go.

7. Cut each wrap in half diagonally and secure with toothpicks if needed.

8. These turkey and avocado wraps are perfect for a quick and satisfying lunch.

Cauliflower Fried Rice

Ingredients:

- 1 small head cauliflower, grated or processed into rice-like consistency
- 1 tablespoon olive oil
- 1/2 cup diced carrots
- 1/2 cup frozen peas
- 2 cloves garlic, minced
- 2 green onions, thinly sliced
- 2 tablespoons low-sodium soy sauce
- 1 tablespoon sesame oil
- 2 eggs, beaten (optional for added protein)

- Salt and pepper to taste

Instructions:

1. Heat the olive oil in a large skillet or wok over medium heat.
2. Add the diced carrots and cook for 2-3 minutes until slightly softened.
3. Stir in the frozen peas, minced garlic, and sliced green onions. Cook for another 2 minutes.
4. Push the vegetables to one side of the skillet and add the beaten eggs to the other side. Scramble the eggs until cooked through.
5. Combine the cooked eggs with the vegetables.
6. Add the grated cauliflower to the skillet and stir to combine with the vegetable and egg mixture.
7. Drizzle the soy sauce and sesame oil over the cauliflower rice. Stir well to coat evenly.
8. Cook for an additional 5 minutes until the cauliflower is tender.
9. Season with salt and pepper to taste.
10. Serve this flavorful and low-carb cauliflower fried rice as a satisfying lunch alternative.

Tuna Salad Lettuce Wraps

Ingredients:

- 2 cans tuna in water, drained
- 1/4 cup diced celery
- 1/4 cup diced red onion
- 2 tablespoons plain Greek yogurt
- 1 tablespoon lemon juice
- 1 tablespoon chopped fresh dill (optional)
- Salt and pepper to taste
- 4 large lettuce leaves (such as romaine or butter lettuce)

Instructions:

1. In a medium bowl, combine the drained tuna, diced celery, diced red onion, Greek yogurt, lemon juice, chopped dill, salt, and pepper. Mix well.
2. Lay out the lettuce leaves on a clean surface.
3. Spoon the tuna salad mixture onto each lettuce leaf.
4. Roll up the lettuce leaves, enclosing the filling.
5. Secure with toothpicks if necessary.
6. These tuna salad lettuce wraps are light, refreshing, and packed with protein.

Lentil Soup with Vegetables

Ingredients:

- 1 cup dried green or brown lentils
- 4 cups low-sodium vegetable broth
- 1 onion, diced
- 2 carrots, diced
- 2 celery stalks, diced
- 2 cloves garlic, minced
- 1 teaspoon dried thyme
- 1 teaspoon dried oregano
- 1 bay leaf
- Salt and pepper to taste
- Fresh parsley for garnish

Instructions:

1. Rinse the lentils under cold water and drain.
2. In a large pot, heat a tablespoon of olive oil over medium heat.
3. Add the diced onion, carrots, celery, and minced garlic to the pot. Sauté for about 5 minutes until the vegetables begin to soften.

4. Add the lentils, vegetable broth, dried thyme, dried oregano, and bay leaf to the pot.

5. Bring the mixture to a boil, then reduce the heat to low and simmer for about 30-40 minutes until the lentils are tender.

6. Season with salt and pepper to taste.

7. Remove the bay leaf before serving.

8. Garnish with fresh parsley.

9. This hearty lentil soup with vegetables is a nutritious and satisfying lunch option.

Mediterranean Chickpea Salad

Ingredients:

- 2 cups canned chickpeas, rinsed and drained
- 1 cup diced cucumber
- 1 cup diced cherry tomatoes
- 1/4 cup diced red onion
- 1/4 cup chopped Kalamata olives
- 1/4 cup crumbled feta cheese
- 2 tablespoons chopped fresh parsley
- Juice of 1 lemon
- 2 tablespoons olive oil

- 1 clove garlic, minced
- Salt and pepper to taste

Instructions:

1. In a large bowl, combine the chickpeas, diced cucumber, diced cherry tomatoes, diced red onion, chopped Kalamata olives, crumbled feta cheese, and chopped fresh parsley.
2. In a small bowl, whisk together the lemon juice, olive oil, minced garlic, salt, and pepper to make the dressing.
3. Pour the dressing over the chickpea salad and toss to combine.
4. Let the salad sit for about 10-15 minutes to allow the flavors to meld together.
5. Serve this vibrant and protein-rich Mediterranean chickpea salad as a refreshing lunch choice.

Greek Chicken Pita Pocket

Ingredients:

- 2 boneless, skinless chicken breasts
- 4 whole wheat pita pockets

- 1/2 cup plain Greek yogurt
- 1 tablespoon lemon juice
- 1 teaspoon dried oregano
- 1 clove garlic, minced
- 1 cup diced cucumber
- 1/2 cup diced tomatoes
- 1/4 cup diced red onion
- 1/4 cup chopped fresh parsley
- Salt and pepper to taste

Instructions:

1. Preheat the grill or stovetop grill pan to medium-high heat.
2. Season the chicken breasts with salt, pepper, and dried oregano.
3. Grill the chicken for about 6-8 minutes per side or until cooked through. Let it rest for a few minutes, then slice it into strips.
4. In a small bowl, combine the Greek yogurt, lemon juice, minced garlic, salt, and pepper to make the yogurt sauce.

5. Warm the whole wheat pita pockets in the oven or on the stovetop.

6. Fill each pita pocket with sliced grilled chicken, diced cucumber, diced tomatoes, diced red onion, and chopped fresh parsley.

7. Drizzle the yogurt sauce over the filling.

8. These Greek chicken pita pockets are a delicious and protein-packed lunch option.

Caprese Skewers with Balsamic Glaze

Ingredients:

- 1 cup cherry tomatoes
- 1 cup small mozzarella balls (bocconcini)
- Fresh basil leaves
- Balsamic glaze
- Salt and pepper to taste

Instructions:

1. Thread a cherry tomato, a mozzarella ball, and a fresh basil leaf onto each skewer.

2. Repeat the process until all the ingredients are used.

3. Arrange the skewers on a serving platter.

4. Drizzle the caprese skewers with balsamic glaze.

5. Sprinkle with salt and pepper to taste.

6. These caprese skewers make for a light and flavorful lunchtime snack.

Shrimp and Veggie Stir-Fry

Ingredients:

- 1 pound shrimp, peeled and deveined
- 2 cups mixed stir-fry vegetables (such as bell peppers, broccoli, snap peas, and carrots)
- 2 cloves garlic, minced
- 2 tablespoons low-sodium soy sauce
- 1 tablespoon sesame oil
- 1 tablespoon honey (optional, or use a sugar substitute for a sugar-free option)
- Salt and pepper to taste

Instructions:

1. Heat the sesame oil in a large skillet or wok over medium-high heat.

2. Add the minced garlic and stir-fry for about 30
   seconds until fragrant.

3. Add the shrimp to the skillet and cook for 2-3
   minutes until they turn pink and opaque.

4. Add the stir-fry vegetables to the skillet and cook
   for an additional 3-4 minutes until they are tender-
   crisp.

5. In a small bowl, whisk together the low-sodium soy
   sauce and honey. Pour the sauce over the shrimp
   and vegetables in the skillet.

6. Stir-fry for another minute to coat the ingredients
   evenly.

7. Season with salt and pepper to taste.

8. This quick and flavorful shrimp and veggie stir-fry
   is a healthy lunch option that is packed with protein
   and vegetables.

Chapter 4: Dinner Recipes

Baked Salmon with Roasted Vegetables

Ingredients:

- 4 salmon fillets
- 1 pound of mixed vegetables (such as bell peppers, zucchini, and broccoli)
- 2 tablespoons of olive oil
- Salt and pepper to taste
- 1 teaspoon of dried herbs (such as thyme or rosemary)

Instructions:

1. Preheat the oven to 400°F (200°C).
2. Place the salmon fillets on a baking sheet lined with parchment paper.
3. In a large bowl, toss the mixed vegetables with olive oil, salt, pepper, and dried herbs.
4. Arrange the seasoned vegetables around the salmon fillets on the baking sheet.

5. Bake in the preheated oven for 15-20 minutes, or until the salmon is cooked through and the vegetables are tender.

6. Serve the baked salmon with roasted vegetables hot and enjoy!

Chicken and Vegetable Stir-Fry

Ingredients:

- 2 boneless, skinless chicken breasts, sliced into thin strips
- 2 cups of mixed vegetables (such as bell peppers, snap peas, and carrots)
- 2 tablespoons of soy sauce (reduced-sodium)
- 1 tablespoon of sesame oil
- 1 tablespoon of minced garlic
- 1 tablespoon of grated ginger
- Salt and pepper to taste

Instructions:

1. Heat sesame oil in a large skillet or wok over medium-high heat.

2. Add the chicken strips and cook until they are browned and cooked through.

3. Add the mixed vegetables to the skillet and stir-fry for 3-4 minutes, or until they are crisp-tender.

4. In a small bowl, whisk together soy sauce, minced garlic, grated ginger, salt, and pepper.

5. Pour the sauce over the chicken and vegetables in the skillet.

6. Stir-fry for an additional 2 minutes, ensuring everything is well coated in the sauce.

7. Remove from heat and serve the chicken and vegetable stir-fry hot.

Turkey Meatballs with Zucchini Noodles

Ingredients:

- 1 pound of ground turkey
- 1/2 cup of whole wheat breadcrumbs
- 1/4 cup of grated Parmesan cheese
- 1/4 cup of chopped fresh parsley
- 1 egg
- 2 cloves of garlic, minced

- 1/2 teaspoon of dried oregano
- Salt and pepper to taste
- 4 medium zucchini, spiralized into noodles
- 1 cup of marinara sauce

Instructions:

1. Preheat the oven to 375°F (190°C).
2. In a large bowl, combine ground turkey, breadcrumbs, Parmesan cheese, parsley, egg, minced garlic, dried oregano, salt, and pepper.
3. Mix the ingredients until well combined.
4. Shape the mixture into meatballs of your desired size.
5. Place the meatballs on a baking sheet lined with parchment paper.
6. Bake in the preheated oven for 20-25 minutes, or until the meatballs are cooked through and browned.
7. While the meatballs are baking, heat the marinara sauce in a skillet over medium heat.

8. Add the spiralized zucchini noodles to the skillet and cook for 2-3 minutes, or until they are slightly softened.

9. Serve the turkey meatballs with zucchini noodles and marinara sauce.

Stuffed Bell Peppers with Quinoa and Ground Turkey

Ingredients:

- 4 bell peppers (any color), tops removed and seeds removed
- 1 pound of ground turkey
- 1 cup of cooked quinoa
- 1/2 cup of diced onion
- 1/2 cup of diced tomatoes
- 1/4 cup of chopped fresh parsley
- 1 clove of garlic, minced
- 1 teaspoon of dried Italian seasoning
- Salt and pepper to taste
- 1/2 cup of shredded mozzarella cheese (optional)

Instructions:

1. Preheat the oven to 375°F (190°C).

2. In a large skillet, cook the ground turkey over medium heat until browned and cooked through.

3. Add the diced onion, diced tomatoes, minced garlic, dried Italian seasoning, salt, and pepper to the skillet.

4. Cook for an additional 3-4 minutes, or until the vegetables are softened.

5. Stir in the cooked quinoa and chopped fresh parsley.

6. Stuff the mixture into the hollowed bell peppers, packing it tightly.

7. Place the stuffed bell peppers in a baking dish and cover with aluminum foil.

8. Bake in the preheated oven for 25-30 minutes, or until the peppers are tender.

9. Remove the foil, sprinkle shredded mozzarella cheese on top (optional), and bake for an additional 5 minutes, or until the cheese is melted and golden.

10. Serve the stuffed bell peppers with quinoa and ground turkey hot.

Baked Cod with Lemon and Herbs

Ingredients:

- 4 cod fillets
- 2 tablespoons of olive oil
- 2 tablespoons of fresh lemon juice
- 2 cloves of garlic, minced
- 1 teaspoon of dried dill
- Salt and pepper to taste
- Lemon slices for garnish

Instructions:

1. Preheat the oven to 400°F (200°C).
2. Place the cod fillets in a baking dish lightly coated with olive oil or lined with parchment paper.
3. In a small bowl, whisk together olive oil, lemon juice, minced garlic, dried dill, salt, and pepper.
4. Drizzle the mixture over the cod fillets, ensuring they are evenly coated.
5. Place lemon slices on top of each fillet for added flavor.
6. Bake in the preheated oven for 12-15 minutes, or until the cod is opaque and flakes easily with a fork.

7. Serve the baked cod with lemon and herbs hot and garnish with additional lemon slices.

Beef and Broccoli Skillet

Ingredients:

- 1 pound of lean beef steak, thinly sliced
- 2 cups of broccoli florets
- 1/4 cup of low-sodium soy sauce
- 2 tablespoons of oyster sauce
- 1 tablespoon of cornstarch
- 1 tablespoon of sesame oil
- 1 tablespoon of minced garlic
- 1 teaspoon of grated ginger
- 1/4 cup of beef broth
- 1 tablespoon of vegetable oil
- Salt and pepper to taste

Instructions:

1. In a small bowl, whisk together soy sauce, oyster sauce, cornstarch, sesame oil, minced garlic, grated ginger, beef broth, salt, and pepper. Set aside.

2. Heat vegetable oil in a large skillet or wok over high heat.

3. Add the thinly sliced beef to the skillet and cook until browned.

4. Remove the beef from the skillet and set aside.

5. In the same skillet, add the broccoli florets and stir-fry for 2-3 minutes, or until they are crisp-tender.

6. Return the beef to the skillet and pour the sauce mixture over the beef and broccoli.

7. Stir-fry for an additional 2 minutes, or until the sauce thickens and coats the beef and broccoli.

8. Remove from heat and serve the beef and broccoli skillet hot.

Eggplant Parmesan with Whole Wheat Pasta

Ingredients:

- 2 large eggplants, sliced into 1/4-inch thick rounds
- 2 cups of marinara sauce
- 1 cup of whole wheat breadcrumbs
- 1/2 cup of grated Parmesan cheese
- 2 eggs, beaten

- 1 teaspoon of dried basil

- 1 teaspoon of dried oregano

- 1/2 teaspoon of garlic powder

- Salt and pepper to taste

- 1/4 cup of chopped fresh basil for garnish (optional)

- Whole wheat pasta, cooked according to package instructions

Instructions:

1. Preheat the oven to 375°F (190°C).

2. In a shallow dish, combine whole wheat breadcrumbs, grated Parmesan cheese, dried basil, dried oregano, garlic powder, salt, and pepper.

3. Dip each eggplant slice into the beaten eggs, allowing excess egg to drip off.

4. Coat the eggplant slice in the breadcrumb mixture, pressing gently to adhere.

5. Place the coated eggplant slices on a baking sheet lined with parchment paper.

6. Bake in the preheated oven for 15-20 minutes, or until the eggplant is golden and crispy.

7. In a baking dish, spread a thin layer of marinara sauce.

8. Arrange a layer of baked eggplant slices on top of the sauce.

9. Continue layering sauce and eggplant until all the ingredients are used, finishing with a layer of sauce on top.

10. Sprinkle grated Parmesan cheese on top (optional).

11. Bake in the oven for 20-25 minutes, or until the sauce is bubbly and the cheese is melted.

12. Garnish with chopped fresh basil (optional) and serve the eggplant Parmesan with whole wheat pasta.

Grilled Shrimp with Garlic and Herbs

Ingredients:

- 1 pound of large shrimp, peeled and deveined
- 2 tablespoons of olive oil
- 2 tablespoons of fresh lemon juice
- 2 cloves of garlic, minced
- 1 tablespoon of chopped fresh parsley
- 1 teaspoon of dried thyme

- Salt and pepper to taste

Instructions:

1. In a bowl, whisk together olive oil, lemon juice, minced garlic, chopped fresh parsley, dried thyme, salt, and pepper.
2. Add the shrimp to the bowl and toss to coat them in the marinade.
3. Cover the bowl and let the shrimp marinate in the refrigerator for 15-30 minutes.
4. Preheat the grill to medium-high heat.
5. Thread the marinated shrimp onto skewers.
6. Grill the shrimp skewers for 2-3 minutes per side, or until they are pink and opaque.
7. Remove from the grill and serve the grilled shrimp with garlic and herbs hot.

Vegetarian Chili with Quinoa

Ingredients:

- 1 cup of quinoa, rinsed
- 1 tablespoon of olive oil
- 1 onion, diced

- 2 cloves of garlic, minced
- 1 bell pepper, diced
- 1 zucchini, diced
- 1 carrot, diced
- 1 can (15 ounces) of kidney beans, drained and rinsed
- 1 can (15 ounces) of black beans, drained and rinsed
- 1 can (15 ounces) of diced tomatoes
- 1 can (6 ounces) of tomato paste
- 2 cups of vegetable broth
- 2 teaspoons of chili powder
- 1 teaspoon of cumin
- Salt and pepper to taste
- Optional toppings: shredded cheese, chopped fresh cilantro, sour cream

Instructions:

1. In a saucepan, cook the quinoa according to the package instructions. Set aside.
2. Heat olive oil in a large pot over medium heat.
3. Add the diced onion and minced garlic to the pot and cook until the onion is translucent and fragrant.

4. Add the diced bell pepper, diced zucchini, and diced carrot to the pot. Cook for 5-7 minutes, or until the vegetables are slightly softened.

5. Stir in the kidney beans, black beans, diced tomatoes, tomato paste, vegetable broth, chili powder, cumin, salt, and pepper.

6. Bring the chili to a boil, then reduce the heat and simmer for 20-30 minutes, allowing the flavors to meld together.

7. Stir in the cooked quinoa and simmer for an additional 5 minutes.

8. Remove from heat and serve the vegetarian chili with quinoa hot.

9. Garnish with shredded cheese, chopped fresh cilantro, and sour cream if desired.

Lemon Herb Grilled Chicken Breast

Ingredients:

- 4 boneless, skinless chicken breasts
- 2 tablespoons of olive oil
- 2 tablespoons of fresh lemon juice
- 2 cloves of garlic, minced

- 1 tablespoon of chopped fresh parsley
- 1 teaspoon of dried thyme
- Salt and pepper to taste

Instructions:

1. In a bowl, whisk together olive oil, lemon juice, minced garlic, chopped fresh parsley, dried thyme, salt, and pepper.
2. Place the chicken breasts in a shallow dish and pour the marinade over them.
3. Cover the dish and let the chicken marinate in the refrigerator for at least 30 minutes, or up to 24 hours for maximum flavor.
4. Preheat the grill to medium-high heat.
5. Remove the chicken breasts from the marinade and discard the remaining marinade.
6. Grill the chicken breasts for 6-8 minutes per side, or until they are cooked through and reach an internal temperature of 165°F (74°C).
7. Remove from the grill and let the chicken rest for a few minutes before serving.
8. Serve the lemon herb grilled chicken breast hot.

Chapter 5: Snacks and Appetizers

These snacks and appetizers are perfect for satisfying cravings while maintaining a healthy diabetic-friendly diet. Enjoy their flavors, textures, and nourishing qualities!

Guacamole with Veggie Sticks

Ingredients:

- 2 ripe avocados
- 1 small onion, finely diced
- 1 tomato, diced
- 1 jalapeno pepper, seeded and minced
- 2 tablespoons fresh cilantro, chopped
- 1 tablespoon lime juice
- Salt and pepper, to taste
- Assorted fresh veggies (carrot sticks, celery sticks, bell pepper slices) for serving

Instructions:

1. Cut the avocados in half, remove the pits, and scoop out the flesh into a bowl.

2. Mash the avocados using a fork until smooth but still slightly chunky.

3. Add the diced onion, tomato, jalapeno pepper, cilantro, lime juice, salt, and pepper to the bowl. Mix well to combine.

4. Taste and adjust the seasoning if needed.

5. Serve the guacamole with veggie sticks for dipping. Enjoy!

Oven-Baked Sweet Potato Fries

Ingredients:

- 2 large sweet potatoes
- 2 tablespoons olive oil
- 1 teaspoon paprika
- 1/2 teaspoon garlic powder
- 1/2 teaspoon salt
- 1/4 teaspoon black pepper

Instructions:

1. Preheat your oven to 425°F (220°C) and line a baking sheet with parchment paper.

2. Peel the sweet potatoes and cut them into thin fry-like strips.

3. In a large bowl, toss the sweet potato strips with olive oil, paprika, garlic powder, salt, and black pepper until evenly coated.

4. Arrange the seasoned sweet potato fries in a single layer on the prepared baking sheet.

5. Bake for 20-25 minutes, flipping halfway through, until the fries are crispy and golden brown.

6. Remove from the oven and let them cool slightly before serving. Enjoy the deliciously healthy sweet potato fries!

Spicy Roasted Chickpeas

Ingredients:

- 2 cups cooked chickpeas (or 1 can, drained and rinsed)
- 1 tablespoon olive oil
- 1 teaspoon paprika
- 1/2 teaspoon cayenne pepper (adjust to your spice preference)
- 1/2 teaspoon garlic powder

- 1/2 teaspoon salt

Instructions:

1. Preheat your oven to 400°F (200°C) and line a baking sheet with parchment paper.

2. In a bowl, combine the chickpeas, olive oil, paprika, cayenne pepper, garlic powder, and salt. Toss until the chickpeas are evenly coated with the spices.

3. Spread the seasoned chickpeas in a single layer on the prepared baking sheet.

4. Roast in the oven for 30-35 minutes, stirring once or twice, until the chickpeas are crispy and slightly golden.

5. Remove from the oven and let them cool before enjoying the spicy roasted chickpeas as a crunchy snack.

Greek Yogurt Dip with Fresh Veggies

Ingredients:

- 1 cup Greek yogurt
- 1 tablespoon fresh lemon juice

- 1 tablespoon fresh dill, chopped
- 1 clove garlic, minced
- Salt and pepper, to taste
- Assorted fresh veggies (carrot sticks, cucumber slices, cherry tomatoes) for dipping

Instructions:

1. In a bowl, combine the Greek yogurt, lemon juice, fresh dill, minced garlic, salt, and pepper. Mix well to incorporate all the flavors.
2. Taste the dip and adjust the seasoning according to your preference.
3. Transfer the Greek yogurt dip to a serving bowl.
4. Arrange the fresh veggies around the dip bowl and serve. Dip the vegetables in the flavorful yogurt dip and enjoy the healthy snack!

Tomato and Mozzarella Skewers

Ingredients:

- Cherry tomatoes
- Fresh mozzarella balls
- Fresh basil leaves

- Balsamic glaze (store-bought or homemade)

Instructions:

1. Take a skewer and thread a cherry tomato onto it, followed by a fresh mozzarella ball and a basil leaf.

2. Repeat the process until you have the desired number of skewers.

3. Drizzle the tomato and mozzarella skewers with balsamic glaze.

4. Arrange the skewers on a platter and serve as an appetizer or snack. Enjoy the delightful combination of flavors!

Baked Parmesan Zucchini Chips

Ingredients:

- 2 medium zucchinis, sliced into thin rounds
- 1/4 cup grated Parmesan cheese
- 1/4 cup breadcrumbs
- 1/2 teaspoon garlic powder
- 1/2 teaspoon dried oregano
- Salt and pepper, to taste
- Olive oil cooking spray

Instructions:

1. Preheat your oven to 425°F (220°C) and line a baking sheet with parchment paper.

2. In a bowl, combine the grated Parmesan cheese, breadcrumbs, garlic powder, dried oregano, salt, and pepper.

3. Dip each zucchini round into the Parmesan mixture, pressing gently to adhere the coating to both sides.

4. Place the coated zucchini rounds on the prepared baking sheet in a single layer.

5. Lightly spray the zucchini rounds with olive oil cooking spray.

6. Bake for 15-20 minutes, or until the zucchini chips are golden and crispy.

7. Allow them to cool slightly before serving. Enjoy the flavorful and guilt-free baked Parmesan zucchini chips!

Hummus with Whole Wheat Pita Bread

Ingredients:

- 1 can chickpeas, drained and rinsed

- 2 tablespoons tahini

- 2 tablespoons lemon juice

- 2 cloves garlic, minced

- 2 tablespoons olive oil

- Salt and cumin, to taste

- Whole wheat pita bread, cut into triangles, for serving

Instructions:

1. In a food processor, combine the chickpeas, tahini, lemon juice, minced garlic, olive oil, salt, and cumin. Process until smooth and creamy.

2. Taste the hummus and adjust the seasoning if needed.

3. Transfer the hummus to a serving bowl and drizzle with a little olive oil.

4. Serve the hummus with whole wheat pita bread triangles. Dip the pita bread into the hummus and savor the delectable flavors.

Caprese Salad Skewers

Ingredients:

- Cherry tomatoes
- Fresh mozzarella balls
- Fresh basil leaves
- Balsamic glaze (store-bought or homemade)

Instructions:

1. Take a skewer and thread a cherry tomato onto it, followed by a fresh mozzarella ball and a basil leaf.
2. Repeat the process until you have the desired number of skewers.
3. Drizzle the tomato, mozzarella, and basil skewers with balsamic glaze.
4. Arrange the skewers on a platter and serve as an appetizer or snack. Enjoy the delightful combination of flavors!

Cottage Cheese and Fresh Berries

Ingredients:

- 1 cup cottage cheese

- Assorted fresh berries (strawberries, blueberries, raspberries)

- Honey or stevia (optional), for drizzling

Instructions:

1. In a bowl, place the cottage cheese.

2. Top the cottage cheese with fresh berries.

3. Drizzle with a little honey or sprinkle with stevia, if desired, for added sweetness.

4. Gently mix the cottage cheese and fresh berries together.

5. Serve the cottage cheese and fresh berries as a refreshing and protein-packed snack.

Antipasto Skewers with Olives and Cheese

Ingredients:

- Cherry tomatoes

- Fresh mozzarella balls

- Sliced salami

- Pitted Kalamata olives

- Fresh basil leaves

- Balsamic glaze (store-bought or homemade)

Instructions:

1. Take a skewer and thread a cherry tomato onto it, followed by a fresh mozzarella ball, a slice of salami, a pitted Kalamata olive, and a basil leaf.

2. Repeat the process until you have the desired number of skewers.

3. Drizzle the antipasto skewers with balsamic glaze.

4. Arrange the skewers on a platter and serve as a flavorful and satisfying appetizer. Enjoy the Mediterranean-inspired combination of ingredients!

Chapter 6: Desserts

Mixed Berry Crisp

Ingredients:

- 2 cups mixed berries (strawberries, blueberries, raspberries)
- 1 tablespoon lemon juice
- 2 tablespoons granulated sweetener (sugar substitute)
- 1/2 cup oats
- 1/4 cup almond flour
- 2 tablespoons unsalted butter, melted
- 1/4 teaspoon cinnamon

Instructions:

1. Preheat the oven to 350°F (175°C).
2. In a bowl, toss the mixed berries with lemon juice and 1 tablespoon of the granulated sweetener.
3. In a separate bowl, combine oats, almond flour, melted butter, remaining granulated sweetener, and cinnamon. Mix well until crumbly.

4. Spread the berry mixture evenly in a baking dish and sprinkle the oat mixture over the top.

5. Bake for 25-30 minutes or until the topping turns golden brown and the berries are bubbling.

6. Remove from the oven and let it cool for a few minutes before serving. Enjoy!

Sugar-Free Chocolate Mousse

Ingredients:

- 1 cup heavy cream
- 1/4 cup unsweetened cocoa powder
- 2 tablespoons powdered sweetener (sugar substitute)
- 1 teaspoon vanilla extract

Instructions:

1. In a mixing bowl, combine heavy cream, cocoa powder, powdered sweetener, and vanilla extract.

2. Using an electric mixer, beat the mixture on medium-high speed until stiff peaks form.

3. Spoon the chocolate mousse into individual serving dishes or glasses.

4. Refrigerate for at least 2 hours to allow the mousse
    to set.

5. Serve chilled and garnish with a sprinkle of cocoa
    powder, if desired.

Baked Apples with Cinnamon and Walnuts

Ingredients:

- 2 medium apples (Granny Smith or Honeycrisp), cored and halved
- 2 tablespoons chopped walnuts
- 1 tablespoon granulated sweetener (sugar substitute)
- 1/2 teaspoon ground cinnamon
- 1 tablespoon unsalted butter, melted

Instructions:

1. Preheat the oven to 375°F (190°C).
2. Place the apple halves in a baking dish, cut side up.
3. In a small bowl, combine chopped walnuts, granulated sweetener, cinnamon, and melted butter.
4. Spoon the walnut mixture into the hollowed-out center of each apple half.

5. Bake for 20-25 minutes or until the apples are tender and the topping is golden brown.

6. Remove from the oven and let them cool slightly before serving. Enjoy!

Greek Yogurt Popsicles

Ingredients:

- 1 cup plain Greek yogurt
- 1/4 cup powdered sweetener (sugar substitute)
- 1 teaspoon vanilla extract
- 1 cup mixed fresh berries (strawberries, blueberries, raspberries)

Instructions:

1. In a bowl, mix together Greek yogurt, powdered sweetener, and vanilla extract until well combined.

2. Gently fold in the mixed fresh berries.

3. Pour the mixture into popsicle molds or small paper cups.

4. Insert popsicle sticks into the molds and freeze for at least 4 hours or until firm.

5. To remove the popsicles from the molds, briefly run them under warm water.

6. Enjoy these refreshing Greek yogurt popsicles on a hot day!

Almond Flour Chocolate Chip Cookies

Ingredients:

- 1 1/2 cups almond flour
- 1/4 cup unsalted butter, softened
- 1/4 cup powdered sweetener (sugar substitute)
- 1/4 cup sugar-free chocolate chips
- 1/2 teaspoon baking powder
- 1/4 teaspoon salt
- 1 teaspoon vanilla extract
- 1 large egg

Instructions:

1. Preheat the oven to 350°F (175°C) and line a baking sheet with parchment paper.

2. In a mixing bowl, cream together softened butter, powdered sweetener, and vanilla extract.

3. Add the egg and mix until well combined.

4. In a separate bowl, whisk together almond flour, baking powder, and salt.

5. Gradually add the dry ingredients to the wet ingredients, mixing until a cookie dough forms.

6. Fold in the sugar-free chocolate chips.

7. Scoop tablespoon-sized portions of dough onto the prepared baking sheet, spacing them apart.

8. Flatten each cookie slightly with the back of a spoon.

9. Bake for 12-15 minutes or until the edges turn golden brown.

10. Remove from the oven and let the cookies cool on the baking sheet for a few minutes before transferring them to a wire rack to cool completely.

Fresh Fruit Salad with Citrus Dressing

Ingredients:

- 2 cups mixed fresh fruit (strawberries, grapes, oranges, pineapple, etc.), chopped or sliced
- 2 tablespoons freshly squeezed orange juice

- 1 tablespoon freshly squeezed lemon juice
- 1 tablespoon honey or powdered sweetener (sugar substitute)
- 1/2 teaspoon grated lemon zest
- Fresh mint leaves for garnish (optional)

Instructions:

1. In a large bowl, combine the mixed fresh fruit.
2. In a separate small bowl, whisk together orange juice, lemon juice, honey or powdered sweetener, and lemon zest to make the citrus dressing.
3. Pour the dressing over the fruit and gently toss until well coated.
4. Refrigerate for at least 30 minutes to allow the flavors to meld together.
5. Garnish with fresh mint leaves before serving. Enjoy this refreshing fruit salad!

Pumpkin Spice Chia Pudding

Ingredients:

- 1/4 cup chia seeds
- 1 cup unsweetened almond milk

- 1/4 cup pumpkin puree

- 1 tablespoon powdered sweetener (sugar substitute)

- 1/2 teaspoon pumpkin pie spice

- 1/2 teaspoon vanilla extract

- Optional toppings: chopped nuts, pumpkin seeds, or cinnamon

Instructions:

1. In a bowl, whisk together chia seeds, almond milk, pumpkin puree, powdered sweetener, pumpkin pie spice, and vanilla extract.

2. Let the mixture sit for 5 minutes, then whisk again to break up any clumps.

3. Cover the bowl and refrigerate for at least 2 hours or overnight.

4. Stir the chia pudding before serving to distribute the seeds evenly.

5. Serve in individual bowls or jars and top with chopped nuts, pumpkin seeds, or a sprinkle of cinnamon if desired.

Peanut Butter Energy Balls

Ingredients:

- 1 cup old-fashioned oats
- 1/2 cup natural peanut butter
- 1/4 cup honey or sugar-free syrup
- 1/4 cup ground flaxseed
- 1/4 cup mini chocolate chips
- 1 teaspoon vanilla extract
- Pinch of salt

Instructions:

1. In a mixing bowl, combine oats, peanut butter, honey or sugar-free syrup, ground flaxseed, chocolate chips, vanilla extract, and salt.
2. Stir well until all the ingredients are evenly incorporated.
3. Place the bowl in the refrigerator for 15-30 minutes to chill.
4. Once chilled, roll the mixture into small bite-sized balls, about 1 inch in diameter.
5. Store the energy balls in an airtight container in the refrigerator for up to a week.

6. Enjoy these nutritious and energizing peanut butter energy balls as a snack or on-the-go treat!

Lemon Poppy Seed Muffins (Sugar-Free)

Ingredients:

- 1 1/2 cups almond flour
- 1/4 cup powdered sweetener (sugar substitute)
- 1 tablespoon poppy seeds
- 1/2 teaspoon baking powder
- 1/4 teaspoon salt
- 1/4 cup unsalted butter, melted
- 1/4 cup fresh lemon juice
- 2 tablespoons lemon zest
- 3 large eggs

Instructions:

1. Preheat the oven to 350°F (175°C) and line a muffin tin with paper liners.
2. In a large mixing bowl, combine almond flour, powdered sweetener, poppy seeds, baking powder, and salt.

3. In a separate bowl, whisk together melted butter, lemon juice, lemon zest, and eggs.

4. Pour the wet ingredients into the dry ingredients and stir until well combined.

5. Divide the batter evenly among the muffin cups, filling each about 2/3 full.

6. Bake for 18-20 minutes or until the muffins are golden brown and a toothpick inserted into the center comes out clean.

7. Remove from the oven and let the muffins cool in the tin for a few minutes before transferring them to a wire rack to cool completely.

Berry Parfait with Greek Yogurt

Ingredients:

- 1 cup plain Greek yogurt
- 1 cup mixed berries (strawberries, blueberries, raspberries)
- 1 tablespoon powdered sweetener (sugar substitute)
- 1/4 cup granola (sugar-free or low-sugar)

Instructions:

1. In a bowl, combine Greek yogurt and powdered
    sweetener. Mix well.
2. In a serving glass or bowl, layer the Greek yogurt,
    mixed berries, and granola.
3. Repeat the layers until all the ingredients are used,
    finishing with a dollop of Greek yogurt on top.
4. Garnish with additional berries and a sprinkle of
    granola if desired.
5. Serve immediately and enjoy this delightful and
    nutritious berry parfait.

Chapter 7: Beverages

Desserts don't have to be off-limits for individuals managing diabetes. With a little creativity and the right ingredients, you can enjoy sweet treats while keeping your blood sugar levels in check. This chapter presents a delightful collection of diabetic-friendly desserts that will satisfy your cravings without compromising your health. So, let's dive into these guilt-free delights and indulge in some delicious sweetness!

Green Smoothie with Spinach and Apple

Ingredients:

- 1 cup fresh spinach leaves
- 1 medium apple, cored and diced
- 1/2 ripe banana
- 1/2 cup unsweetened almond milk
- 1/2 cup plain Greek yogurt
- 1 tablespoon chia seeds
- Ice cubes (optional)

Instructions:

1. In a blender, combine the spinach, apple, banana, almond milk, Greek yogurt, and chia seeds.
2. Blend until smooth and creamy.
3. If desired, add ice cubes and blend again until well incorporated.
4. Pour into a glass and serve immediately. Enjoy the refreshing goodness of this green smoothie!

Iced Raspberry Tea

Ingredients:

*   2 cups fresh raspberries
*   4 cups water
*   4 tea bags (black or green tea)
*   Stevia or sugar substitute, to taste
*   Lemon slices for garnish (optional)
*   Ice cubes

Instructions:

1. In a saucepan, combine the raspberries and water. Bring to a boil and let simmer for 5 minutes.

2. Remove from heat and strain the raspberry mixture to remove the seeds.

3. Return the raspberry-infused water to the saucepan and bring it to a boil again.

4. Add the tea bags and steep for the recommended time according to the tea package instructions.

5. Remove the tea bags and stir in the desired amount of stevia or sugar substitute.

6. Let the mixture cool, then refrigerate until chilled.

7. Serve over ice cubes with lemon slices for garnish, if desired. Savor the fruity and refreshing flavors of this iced raspberry tea!

Cucumber and Mint Infused Water

Ingredients:

- 1 large cucumber, thinly sliced
- 10-12 fresh mint leaves
- 8 cups water
- Ice cubes

Instructions:

1. In a large pitcher, combine the cucumber slices and fresh mint leaves.

2. Pour water over the cucumber and mint, ensuring they are fully submerged.

3. Cover the pitcher and refrigerate for at least 2 hours to allow the flavors to infuse.

4. Serve the infused water over ice cubes. Stay hydrated with this cool and rejuvenating cucumber and mint combination!

Homemade Sugar-Free Lemonade

Ingredients:

- 4-5 lemons, juiced
- 4 cups water
- Stevia or sugar substitute, to taste
- Lemon slices for garnish (optional)
- Ice cubes

Instructions:

1. In a pitcher, combine the freshly squeezed lemon juice and water.

2. Add the desired amount of stevia or sugar substitute, adjusting to your preferred level of sweetness.

3. Stir well to dissolve the sweetener.

4. Refrigerate the lemonade until chilled.

5. Serve over ice cubes with lemon slices for garnish, if desired. Enjoy the tangy and refreshing taste of this homemade sugar-free lemonade!

Almond Milk Latte

Ingredients:

- 1 cup unsweetened almond milk
- 1 shot of espresso or 1/2 cup brewed coffee
- Stevia or sugar substitute, to taste
- Ground cinnamon for sprinkling (optional)

Instructions:

1. Heat the almond milk in a small saucepan over low heat until hot but not boiling.

2. In a coffee mug, combine the espresso or brewed coffee and the desired amount of stevia or sugar substitute.

3. Pour the hot almond milk over the coffee mixture, holding back the foam with a spoon.

4. Spoon the milk foam on top.

5. Sprinkle ground cinnamon on top for added flavor, if desired. Savor the creamy and comforting goodness of this almond milk latte!

Strawberry Banana Smoothie

Ingredients:

- 1 cup frozen strawberries
- 1 ripe banana
- 1/2 cup plain Greek yogurt
- 1/2 cup unsweetened almond milk
- 1 tablespoon flaxseeds
- Ice cubes (optional)

Instructions:

1. In a blender, combine the frozen strawberries, banana, Greek yogurt, almond milk, and flaxseeds.

2. Blend until smooth and creamy.

3. If desired, add ice cubes and blend again until well incorporated.

4. Pour into a glass and enjoy this luscious and nutritious strawberry banana smoothie!

Coconut Water Electrolyte Drink

Ingredients:

- 2 cups unsweetened coconut water
- 1/4 cup freshly squeezed orange juice
- 1/4 cup freshly squeezed lime juice
- 2 tablespoons honey or sugar substitute
- Pinch of sea salt
- Ice cubes

Instructions:

1. In a pitcher, combine the coconut water, orange juice, lime juice, honey or sugar substitute, and a pinch of sea salt.
2. Stir well to dissolve the sweetener and salt.
3. Refrigerate until chilled.
4. Serve over ice cubes. Replenish your electrolytes and quench your thirst with this revitalizing coconut water drink!

Sparkling Water with Citrus Slices

Ingredients:

- Sparkling water
- Lemon slices
- Lime slices
- Orange slices
- Ice cubes

Instructions:

1. Fill a glass with sparkling water.
2. Add lemon, lime, and orange slices to the glass.
3. Drop in a few ice cubes for extra chilliness.
4. Stir gently and enjoy the effervescence and tangy flavors of this refreshing sparkling water with citrus slices!

Chai Tea with Almond Milk

Ingredients:

- 2 cups water
- 2 chai tea bags
- 1 cup unsweetened almond milk
- Stevia or sugar substitute, to taste

- Ground cinnamon for sprinkling (optional)

Instructions:

1. In a saucepan, bring the water to a boil.

2. Remove from heat and add the chai tea bags.

3. Let the tea steep for the recommended time according to the tea package instructions.

4. Remove the tea bags and stir in the almond milk.

5. Add the desired amount of stevia or sugar substitute, adjusting to your preferred level of sweetness.

6. Heat the mixture over low heat until hot but not boiling.

7. Pour into mugs and sprinkle ground cinnamon on top, if desired. Savor the aromatic and spiced flavors of this comforting chai tea with almond milk!

Detox Water with Lemon and Ginger

Ingredients:

- 4 cups water
- 1 lemon, thinly sliced

- 1-inch piece of fresh ginger, peeled and thinly sliced
- Fresh mint leaves
- Ice cubes

Instructions:

1. In a pitcher, combine the water, lemon slices, ginger slices, and fresh mint leaves.
2. Stir well to mix the ingredients.
3. Refrigerate for at least 2 hours to allow the flavors to infuse.
4. Serve the detox water over ice cubes. Enjoy the cleansing and invigorating properties of this lemon and ginger detox water!

CONCLUSION

Managing diabetes through a healthy diet is not only essential but also achievable. By incorporating the right ingredients and making mindful choices, we can create meals that are both delicious and beneficial for our well-being. This cookbook has aimed to provide you with a diverse array of recipes that cater to different tastes, ensuring that you never have to compromise on flavor while maintaining a balanced diabetic-friendly diet.

One of the key takeaways from this cookbook is the importance of portion control. Controlling the quantity of food we consume plays a crucial role in managing blood sugar levels. By following the serving sizes indicated in the recipes and being mindful of portion sizes, we can maintain a healthy balance and prevent unnecessary spikes in glucose levels.

Additionally, we have emphasized the significance of choosing whole, unprocessed foods. Fresh fruits, vegetables, lean proteins, and whole grains are rich in essential nutrients and fiber, which can help stabilize blood sugar levels and promote overall well-being. By incorporating these wholesome ingredients into our meals, we nourish our bodies and support optimal health.

Remember, managing diabetes is a lifelong commitment, and the choices we make in the kitchen play a vital role in our overall well-being. By incorporating the recipes and principles outlined in this cookbook into your lifestyle, you are taking a proactive step towards a healthier future.

So, as you embark on your culinary adventures armed with this knowledge, let your kitchen be a space of creativity, nourishment, and enjoyment. May these recipes inspire you to discover new flavors, experiment with ingredients, and create meals that not only support your health but also bring delight to your taste buds.

Thank you for joining us on this journey through the "Super Easy Diabetic Cookbook for Beginners." May your cooking endeavors be filled with deliciousness, good health, and the joy of sharing nourishing meals with loved ones. Here's to a vibrant and fulfilling life as you embrace the power of food in managing diabetes.

Wishing you a future brimming with health, happiness, and culinary exploration.